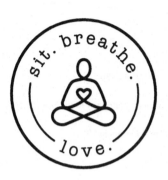

sit. breathe. love.

You are here.

A mindful travel journal

By Emma Clarke

A Sit. Breathe. Love. publication

Sit. Breathe. Love. is an imprint of Identity Withheld Ltd.

First printed in Great Britain in 2014

By Identity Withheld Ltd.

ISBN 978-1-910306-00-0

Cover and interior design by Rebecca Perry
www.rebeccaperrydesign.com

Identity Withheld Ltd's policy is to use papers that are natural,
renewable and recyclable products and made from wood grown in
sustainable forests. The logging and manufacturing processes are
expected to conform to the environmental regulations of the
country of origin.

www.identitywithheld.com

"The real voyage of discovery consists not in seeing new landscapes but in having new eyes."

Marcel Proust

This is your journey.

This is your story.

It starts NOW.

I dedicate this journey to:

....

This could be a person.

It could be a concept.

It could be your future self?

Contents

Reflecting

Mindfulness mʌɪn(d)f(ʊ)lnəs

"Mindfulness can be cultivated by
paying attention in a specific way,
that is in the present moment, and as
non-reactively, non-judgmentally and
open-heartedly as possible."

Dr Jon Kabat-Zinn

Hello.

I'm your journal. I am an analogue antidote to a digital world.

I'm your Ideal Travel Pal. I have no annoying habits. I do not snore.
I never criticise you, moan about your timekeeping, your wardrobe
choices or how and where our time is spent. I never whinge. I never
slurp my tea. I never dribble egg down the front of my T-shirt.
I'm never late for the bus. I will do whatever you want me to do.
No complaints.

One more thing: **I LOVE EVERYTHING YOU DO!**

Seriously. Your life is *amazing* to me.

Everything you write in my pages is all about *you*. I'm a great reason
for you to indulge yourself in some unprecedented *you-time*. Cram
your experiences into me. Pin your moments into me. My empty
pages ache for all the potential your life has to offer.

This is your trip, man.

Flick through me now.

Look at all those pages.

Look at all that *emptiness*. Imagine how *full* my pages yearn to be.

I promise your secrets are safe with me. I won't tell, like, *A SOUL.*
But if someone happens to pick me up and read what's been
written inside me, well... that's outta my hands, clearly.

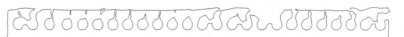

So keep me safe.

What I really want to say is, I'm here for you. No matter where you go or what you do. What you do with your precious time is your business. I'm just here to help you enjoy it as much and for as long as is cosmologically possible.

Me and you: we're a great team. Trust me, I'm a journal.

One more thing: did you bring snacks?

Because I'll level with you – I get cranky if there aren't any snacks.

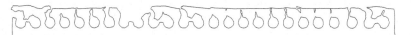

How to use me

1. Write, doodle, glue, scribble, draw and stick stuff all over me. Every last inch of me. My margins, my headers and footers, the cute little road sign icons, the handy doodle boxes, my front and my back. **DEFACE ME, BABY.**

2. Fill me with anything that holds a memory or captures a moment.

3. You don't have to go through the pages in order. What you do and when you do it is up to you.

4. You'll definitely need a roll of sticky tape. A glue stick might work too, although not necessarily for all the activities I'll suggest to you. But really, trust me on the sticky tape.

Have a go now. Go on.

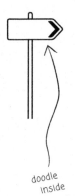

doodle
inside
the sign

How do you feel about starting your Mindful Travel Journal?
Draw a self-portrait to depict how you're feeling right now. **GO!**

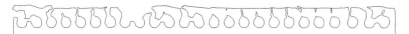

What is mindfulness?

It's a good question. Mindfulness is a subtle so-and-so. Mindfulness means paying deliberate attention to the present moment, with qualities like compassion, acceptance, patience, kindness and curiosity.

Sounds like a lot of hard work? Here's the thing: if you're putting in a lot of effort, it's not mindfulness. Mindfulness is **SIMPLE SIMPLICITY** and it takes very little effort.

Mindfulness is truly a way of being that has the potential to change the way you look at the world and all the elements of your life: your work, your relationships, your finances, your playtime – everything. By practicing mindfulness you can make the present moment a more wonderful place to be. When you're taking a vacation every moment of your holiday time is precious; you probably work really hard and probably don't get much time off. Mindful travel helps you to fully experience every moment of your journey in rich and meaningful ways.

Really, travelling mindfully means you get better value from your holiday.

By paying focused attention on the present you can live more fully, making deliberate choices for every moment of your life. The present moment is the moment you have now; ultimately, it's the only moment you ever have. As soon as you've recognised 'the present' it's become the past because the moment you thought was 'now' has just passed into the past. The future isn't here yet and the past has just happened, so really all we can ever have is now, this present moment.

This journal helps you to put a moment on a page. To identify a thought, a feeling, an insight in a creative way. The act of putting it on the page will help you steady your mind and commit the moment to your memory of mindfulness. Honestly: this is a beautiful process.

It's been said that mindfulness is awareness of the moment 'from the heart.' This means mindfulness practice gives rise to a deep connection from your inner, most true self to the present moment.

It's true that if you change the way you look at things, the things you look at change. And if it's true that what we resist persists, it's also true that what we accept transforms.

This journal gives you an opportunity to transform the way you experience travel.

As you embark upon your mindful travels, be prepared to experience places, people, landscapes – everything – in a fresh new way, every minute of your holiday.

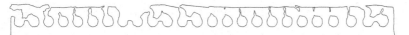

How to cultivate mindfulness

By adopting the seven mindsets described below, you can help your mindfulness practice become a way of being. Regular meditation practice is extremely helpful in developing a mindful attitude, but it's not the only way. To cultivate an attitude of compassionate curiosity towards yourself and the world around you, take time to contemplate every day, whether in deliberate meditation, bungee-jumping, sitting in an airplane seat, swimming, eating lunch (it could be anything you like). Create a mental space where you limit your distractions and focus on your activity.

1. **Non-judging**
   Take the position of an impartial witness to your own experiences. Become aware of your judgmental thoughts (towards either yourself or others) and take a step back. Notice when you slip into categorising people and events into 'good' and 'bad', 'positive' and 'negative.' Try to experience them just as they are, without judgements. Notice how often you become preoccupied with 'liking' or 'disliking' something.

2. **Patience**
   Sometimes things unfold in their own time; you don't get daffodils in December! Practicing mindfulness helps us to experience our own unfolding moment by moment. Why rush on to the next moment when we can experience our life in the one we have now?

3. **Beginner's mind**
   Practicing mindfulness means taking the chance to see everything as if we were seeing it for the very first time. Sometimes the illusion of 'knowing' can prevent us from experiencing our lives now, in the present as they really are

and not how we expect them to be. Try to see something new in people, places, situations that are very familiar. You might experience them in a new, fresh way.

4. Trust

Trusting yourself is a key part of meditation practice. If you can cultivate a calm and peaceful mind to the point where you can honestly trust yourself you can become wholly and truly yourself.

5. Non-striving

Mindfulness and meditation is really about non-doing; it has no goal other than 'being.' If you meditate and practice mindfulness to get relaxed, stress-free, happy and enlightened you'll struggle to succeed. Just let your practice be what it is, experience every moment for what it is and take what you can from every meditation session.

6. Acceptance

Often acceptance comes after we've been through an intense period of stress or turmoil. Sometimes we can't change things but accepting our circumstances means we stop struggling against them, wasting time and energy on thinking about situations that are beyond our control.

7. Letting go

When we pay attention to our inner experience, we discover there are certain thoughts, feelings and situations that our mind wants to hold on to. If it's a pleasant experience, we try and prolong our pleasure; if it's unpleasant we can either dwell on the source of our discomfort or try to forcefully push it away. In meditation, we try to intentionally put aside our tendency to cling onto some aspects of our experience and reject others.

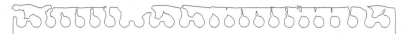

Meditation

There are many different ways to meditate, and as it's such a personal practice there are probably infinite ways to do it. Mindful meditation is where you focus on one specific thing – it could be your breathing, a physical sensation or a particular object outside of you. The purpose of this type of meditation is to focus strongly on one thing and continually and gently bring your attention back to that focus when your mind wanders. (Which it will. A lot).

It's true that focused attention is very much like a muscle; it needs to be strengthened through exercise. And the more we meditate, the less anxiety we have. This is because we're actually loosening the connections of particular neural pathways.

There's a section of our brains that's sometimes referred to as the Me Centre (it's technically the medial prefrontal cortex). This is the part that processes information relating to ourselves and our experiences. Normally the neural pathways from the bodily sensation and fear centres of the brain to the Me Centre are really strong. When you experience a scary or upsetting sensation, it triggers a strong reaction in your Me Centre, making you feel scared and under attack.

When we meditate, we weaken this neural connection. This means that we don't react as strongly to sensations that might have once lit up our Me Centres. As we weaken this connection, we simultaneously strengthen the connection between what's known as our Assessment Centre (the part of our brains known for reasoning) and our bodily sensation and fear centres. So when we experience scary or upsetting sensations, we can more easily look at them rationally and with much less anxiety.

For example, when you experience pain, rather than becoming anxious and assuming it means something is wrong with you, you can watch the pain rise and fall without becoming ensnared in a story about what it might mean.

Scientists have shown that regular meditation can foster more creativity, greater compassion, better memory, less stress and more grey matter.

So meditating is definitely good for you. But how do you do it?

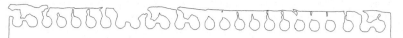

Mindful breathing exercises

Breathing is such a simple practice but it can transform your life. We all breathe and most of the time, we're not even aware of it. With mindful breathing, when you breathe in, know that you're breathing in. When you breathe out, know you're breathing out. The great meditation master Thich Nhat Hanh teaches five simple mindfulness exercises to help you live with happiness and joy.

Mindfulness practice should be enjoyable, and shouldn't take great effort. Breathing in doesn't take much effort and we don't often think about it – we just do it. To breathe in, just breathe in. Simply allow your breath to take place. As you do it, become aware of it and enjoy it, effortlessly.

The same thing is true with walking mindfully. We walk a lot. We don't often think about it. With mindful walking, every step you take is enjoyable. Every step helps you become aware of the wonders of life, in yourself and around you. Every step is a step towards inner peace. Every step is connecting with the earth. Every step is an opportunity to feel joy.

During the time you are practicing mindfulness, you stop talking – not only the talking outside, but the talking inside that constantly goes on in our heads. This internal dialogue goes on and on and on inside you, without you really being conscious of the quality of thoughts that flit across your mind. Real silence is the cessation of talking – of both the mouth and of the mind. This silence isn't oppressive or restrictive. It's a very elegant, powerful kind of silence. It is the kind of silence that heals and nourishes us.

Another source of happiness is concentration. When you are aware of something, such as breathing, walking or even a flower, and can maintain that awareness, your focus is concentrated. When your mindfulness becomes powerful, your concentration becomes powerful, and when you are fully concentrated, you have a chance to make a breakthrough and achieve insight. If you meditate on a cloud, you can get insight into the nature of the cloud. You can meditate on yourself, or negative feelings like anger and fear, or your sense of joy and peace.

Anything can be the object of your meditation – people, places, objects, food, music, art. When your mindfulness and concentration are powerful, your insight will liberate you from fear, anger, and despair, and bring you true joy, true peace, and true happiness.

Mindful breathing

The first exercise is very simple, but the results can be transformative. The exercise is simply to identify the in-breath as the in-breath and the out-breath as the out-breath. When you breathe in, you know that this is your in-breath. When you breathe out, you are mindful that this is your out-breath.

Just recognise: this is an in-breath, this is an out-breath. It really is that simple. In order to recognise your in-breath as in-breath, you have to bring your mind gently 'home' to yourself and your breathing. The object of your mindfulness is your breath, and you just focus your attention on it. Breathing in, this is your in-breath. Breathing out, this is your out-breath. When you do that, the mental chatter will stop. You don't think or follow your own internal dialogue any more. You don't have to make an effort to stop

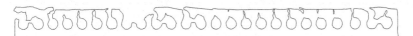

your thinking; you bring your attention to your in-breath and the mental chatter just stops. You don't think of the past any more. You don't think of the future. You just focus your attention, your mindfulness, on your breath.

You are breathing in, and while breathing in, you know that you are alive. The in-breath can be a celebration of the fact that you are alive, so it can be very joyful. When you are joyful and happy, you don't feel that you have to make any effort at all. You are alive; you are breathing in. To be still alive is a miracle. The greatest of all miracles is to be alive, and when you breathe in, you touch that miracle. Therefore, your breathing can be a celebration of life.

An in-breath may take three, four, five seconds, maybe more. That's time to be alive, time to enjoy your breath. You don't have to interfere with your breathing. If your in-breath is short, allow it to be short. If your out-breath is long, let it be long. Don't try to force it. The practice is simple recognition of the in-breath and the out-breath.

Concentration

The second exercise is about concentration – that while you breathe in, you follow your in-breath from the beginning to the end. If your in-breath lasts three or four seconds, then your mindfulness also lasts three or four seconds. From the beginning of your out-breath to the end of your out-breath, your mind is always with it. Therefore, mindfulness becomes uninterrupted, and the quality of your concentration is improved.

So the second exercise is to follow your in-breath and your out-breath all the way through. Whether they are short or long, it doesn't matter. What is important is that you follow your in-breath from the very beginning to the very end. Your awareness is sustained with no interruption. Suppose you are breathing in, and then you think, "Oh, I forgot to send an email." There is an interruption. Just stick to your in-breath all the way through. Then you cultivate your mindfulness and your concentration. You *become* your in-breath. You *become* your out-breath. If you continue like that, your breathing will naturally become deeper and slower, more harmonious and peaceful. You don't have to make any effort – it just happens naturally.

Awareness of your body

The third exercise is to become aware of your body as you are breathing. "Breathing in, I am aware of my whole body." This takes the practice one step further.

In the first exercise, you became aware of your in-breath and your out-breath. Because you have now generated the energy of mindfulness through mindful breathing, you can use that energy to recognise your body.

"Breathing in, I am aware of my body. Breathing out, I am aware of my body." You know your body is there. When your mind is with your body, you are well established in the here and the now. You are fully alive. You can be in touch with the wonders of life that are available in yourself and around you.

This exercise is simple, but the effect of the oneness of body and mind is very great. In our daily lives, we are rarely in that situation. Our body is there but our mind is elsewhere. Our mind gets caught in the past or in the future, in regrets, sorrow, fear, or uncertainty, and

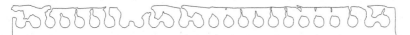

so our mind is not present. Our mind could be off with the future, with our projects, and we're not there for our children or our partner.

When you practice mindful breathing, there is more peace and harmony in your breathing, and if you continue this practice, the peace and the harmony will penetrates into your body, into your being.

Releasing tension

The next exercise is to release the tension in the body. When you are truly aware of your body, you notice there is some tension and pain in your body, some kind of stress. The tension and pain might have been accumulating for a long time and our bodies suffer. We often don't realise how physically tense we are until we focus our minds on noticing it.

It doesn't matter what position you're in – sitting, lying, or standing – it's always possible to release the tension. You can practice total relaxation, deep relaxation, in a sitting or lying position. While you are driving, you might notice the tension in your body, a stiffness in your jaw, neck and shoulders. You are in a hurry and feel stressed about the traffic. When you come to a red light, you're impatient to get moving again. But the red light can be a reminder to try and relax. Take opportunity offered by the red light to practice mindful breathing and release the tension in the body.

So next time you're stopped at a red light, you might like to sit back and practice the fourth exercise: "Breathing in, I'm aware of my body. Breathing out, I release the tension in my body." Peace is possible at that moment, and it can be practiced many times a day – at work, while you are driving, while you are cooking, while you are doing the dishes, while you are walking. It is always possible to practice

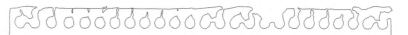

releasing the tension in your body; it follows that when you do that, the tension in your mind eases at the same time.

Walking meditation

When you practice mindful breathing you simply allow your in-breath to take place. You become aware of it and enjoy it without effort. The same thing is true with mindful walking. Every step is enjoyable. Every step helps you touch the wonders of life. Every step is joy.

You don't have to make any effort during walking meditation, because it is so simple, so enjoyable. You are there, body and mind together. You are fully alive, fully present in the here and the now. With every step, you can celebrate the wonder of life and appreciate everything that is around you. When you walk mindfully, every step brings healing. Every step brings peace and joy, because every step is a miracle.

The real miracle is not to fly or walk on fire. The real miracle is to walk on the Earth, and you can perform that miracle at any time. Just bring your mind home to your body, become alive, and perform the joyful miracle of walking on Earth.

To learn more about Thich Nhat Hanh and teachings, we heartily recommend his book 'The Miracle of Mindfulness.'

Your time

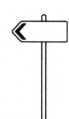

How you spend your time during your travels is your business. As I said: *no judgements*. Even if you rock up drunk in a police cell wearing a clown costume that smells of ponies **IT'S YOUR BUSINESS, HONEY.**

But seriously.

How do you want to spend your time during your travels? Once you've pondered this for a while, you can work out if your choices are helping you develop a calm, peaceful mind... and if they're not, perhaps you can guide yourself to make a different set of choices that will serve you better and help you really enjoy yourself.

How you've previously spent your holiday and travel time...

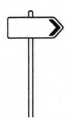 How you want to spend your holiday and travel time now...

Preparing

Your itinerary

Space for departure and return dates, flight numbers, train times, where you're staying, what you've already planned to do when you get there... all the info that's essential to help you get to where you're going. Write it all here so all the info's in one place.

You'll thank me later, sugar.

Space for more trip-of-a-lifetime travel details

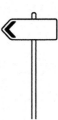

Packing list

Make a list of everything you want to take with you. Pants, phone charger, medicine, passport. You know the kind of thing. (Two key words to bear in mind here: **BAGGAGE ALLOWANCE**).

Space for more packing-type brainstorm doodles.

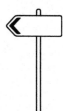

fill the box
with doodles

Things to do before you go

Make a list here of all the things you need to do and get organised before you go on your trip. You might include setting up your email auto-reply, taking out all the stuff out of your fridge that's going to go 'science project' while you're away, asking someone to feed your goldfish... all the stuff you need to get set up so you can empty your head and enjoy your trip.

Things to do to help your body prepare for the trip

Need to have any jabs? Buy some travel sickness bands? Maybe you need to put in some training so you can frolic uphill like a perky mountain goat. Write down all the things you can do to prepare your body for your holiday. (Note: Go easy on yourself. No criticism or metaphorical self-flagellation of your body in any way, shape or form. You're beautiful. Honestly. But hey, if *actual* self-flagellation is your bag, that's **YOUR PRIVATE BUSINESS**).

Your hopes

What do you want to get out of this trip? Why are you going? And heck, why **THERE**?

Wannados

A brain-dump of things you want to do on this trip: places to see, adventures to have, hopes to dream...

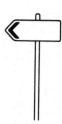

Inspirational quotes and mottos to inspire you on your travels

Space for more inspirational stuff

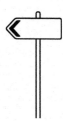

Affirmations

Write some short, positive statements about yourself that you can turn to if you get the travel jitters. (They're usually written in the present tense to anchor you to the glorious, *mindfulicious* here and now). Here are some examples:

"I have an adventurer's sprit and I relish the opportunity to explore the world."

"I trust myself to do the best for myself, all the time."

"I am joyful and curious as I travel and explore the planet."

"I travel in style."

Experiencing

In transit

As you wander through departure lounges, waiting rooms and (usually) the large metal boxes in which we drive, fly or float across the globe from A to B, what do you notice about being in transit? The food, the smells, the décor? And oh my, what about the **PEOPLE**?

Stick an item you picked up on your outward-bound journey here: a serviette, a sweet, a member of the cabin crew – anything.

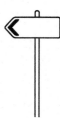

Stick your tickets, boarding cards and seat reservation slips here.

Your accommodation

No-one has ever seen this place in the same way you're seeing it right now, right here, in this moment.

You're the first person to experience this room in quite the way you're doing now. This moment is yours. No-one else is going to be here again at this time, not even you. Enjoy it!

Look around your new temporary home. How would you describe it? What are your first impressions? Slowly walk around it with your eyes closed and your hands outstretched (be careful not to trip! As a journal, I cannot be held legally responsible for small collisions with occasional tables). What do you notice? Use all your senses.

Draw a floorplan or a picture of where you're staying. Or take a pic and stick it here.

Your view

What can you see from your window? Do you even *have* a window?

Remember, no-one has ever looked at this view in the way you are doing now. It's a unique experience for you and the world around you – it's never been looked at like this before.

Write some words that come into your head when you look beyond your room out into the rest of the world.

What can you hear?

What can you smell?

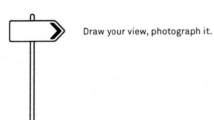

Draw your view, photograph it.

Tastes

Part of the joy of travel is experiencing new food. Isn't it?? (Is it?)

If you're an adventurous mega-foodie or a timid nibbler, scribble all your thoughts about the food you eat on your holiday here.

Stick in wrappers, packaging, even smear ketchup on the page if that helps.

Stick a drinks mat from your favourite bar here.

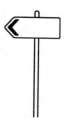

Splodge a 'glass ring' from your favourite holiday drink here. Make a pattern that looks a flower or a bit of sacred geometry if you're in the mood.

Smells

Everywhere smells, right? And sometimes, it has to be said, *not in a good way*. What does your trip **SMELL** like? What evocative olfactory memory will you take away with you?

Spray something glorious on this page.

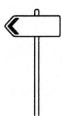

Write some random words that describe what it smells like.

Sights

This could mean pretty much anything: the idyllic mountaintop monastery, the open vista of the desert or that person in the room next door who has unforgettable taste in swimwear. Describe, draw, scribble and doodle your trip's memorable sights here.

Space for more sights.

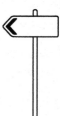

Sounds

Ssh. What can you hear? Distant mopeds? Cowbells? Singing nuns? (Or is that just happening in *my* head??) Really listen to your environment and write down all the sounds you're not used to hearing.

Make up some nonsense words to describe the sounds you can hear.

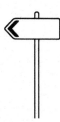

The landscape

You might be in the parched outback, a tropical paradise or a snow-dusted palace surrounded by rocky wonder. Look deeply at all the landscapes you experience on your trip. How will you remember them when you get home?

Go outside and draw a picture of whatever you can see that's straight in front of you. Not to the left. Not to the right. *Directly in front of you.*

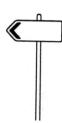

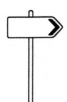

Stick something on this page that will always remind you of this place, this time.

Stick a leaf, a pebble, some sand – anything that represents the landscape in which you're currently living – here. (Tip: use your sticky-tape. Glue would be really rubbish in this circumstance).

Textures

Silky, smooth, damp or squidgy? What textures are you touching on your trip? These might be physical or metaphorical.

And quite literally, *how do you feel?*

Take the rough with the smooth and stick as many different textured things on this page.

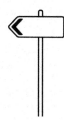

Creatures

You might encounter all sorts of creatures on your travels: insects, jungle animals or the family in the upstairs apartment. Use all your senses to describe the creatures you meet.

Draw a creature you've seen here, or stick in a photo. (Do not stick the actual creature on this page. That would be wrong, wrong, wrong).

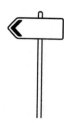

Weather

Are you feeling **HOT**??

The chances are you're witnessing weather that's out of your usual meteorological experience. Describe the climate where you are now. Draw the weather if you're visually inclined.

How does the weather make you feel? What do you notice about the weather and your reaction to it?

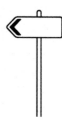

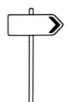

Leave this page open outside for at least a couple of hours or better still, overnight. (Note: Probably best to weigh down and maybe hide your journal so it doesn't blow away or get eaten by wild dogs). WARNING: If it rains, the pages might go a bit, you know, *pulpy*.

Has the weather made any difference to the page?

Your body

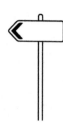

Travel can do all sorts of things to your body. How's your body coping?
(Note: smearing journal pages with matter that has originated inside your body
is potentially **UNWISE**).

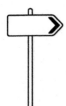

Draw a picture to describe how your body feels on this trip. Stick in some photos if you fancy it: sore feet, a great tan, a tattoo.

Your sleep

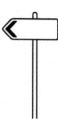

A strange bed, a different time zone, a shift in climate – all these things can alter your sleep pattern. How are you sleeping? How does it feel to sleep in this place?

Anything helping or stopping you from sleeping?

Have you had any crazy dreams? Draw them as a cartoon strip here.

Landmarks

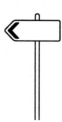

Landmarks don't have to be huge iconic places you see on postcards. You might have your own special *personal* landmarks. Write a list here.

Spend some time at your landmarks, sitting mindfully. What do you notice?

Culture shock

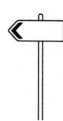

You may be seeing, doing, tasting, hearing, smelling and generally **WITNESSING** things that are definitely outside your comfort zone. Frankly, you may be feeling really quite startled. Put all your culture shocks down here.

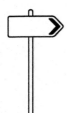

What have you experienced that's broadened your horizons?

People

Travel books and brochures often talk about 'friendly locals' and when travelling
you're inevitably going to meet new people. Who have you met on your trip?
How have they touched you? (Not necessarily in **THAT** way). What idiosyncrasies
do they have?

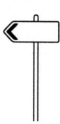

How will you remember the people you've met?

Are you going to keep in touch? If so, write their contact details here.

Beliefs

No matter where you travel – even if it's only round the corner from where you live
– it's possible you'll encounter people who have a very different set of beliefs to
yours. What do you notice about the beliefs of the people where you are now?
Does it inspire you? Is it touching anything inside you? Describe the feeling.

Are any of your own beliefs being challenged by what you're experiencing?

Phrases

This might be foreign phrases you've learned that have helped get you out of trouble or it might be the kind of catchphrases that become a running gag on a trip. Note them down here. They will probably make no sense to anyone else whatsoever.

Think about what these words really mean and how they help your relationships, even with strangers.

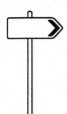 Space for more phrases and buzzwords.

Art

There will be art around you – architecture, paintings, statues, textiles, crafts, music and yes, even folk-dancing. What kind of art are you enjoying? Are your tastes changing?

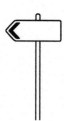

Draw very scientific-looking diagrams of your own versions of the art you've taken pleasure in during your trip.

History

Have you learned some interesting historical facts on your journey? Everyone loves a historical fact or two. (They do, don't they??)

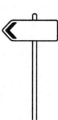

What events from the past have the most meaning for you on this trip?

Trivia

Picked up any curious facts on your travels? Write them here.

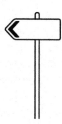

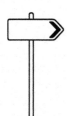

Space for more trivia. You never know, it could come in handy at a Pub Quiz.

Random acts of kindness

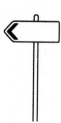

People can be extremely kind and thoughtful. Are you experiencing anything that enhances your faith in human kindness?

The comfort of strangers

One of the best things about travel is that you don't know the people you encounter and you'll probably never see most of them again, ever. Has a stranger offered you comfort? (Of any sort, really. Again, nobody's judging here...)

Space for more comfort from strangers.

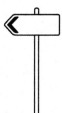

Eavesdropping

Listening in to other people's conversations might be morally dubious but sometimes it's unavoidable. (Especially, in my experience, in confined spaces. If you're doing it right now, for goodness' sake, be discreet!). Have you unwittingly overheard any gems you want to remember for posterity?

Space for more overheard nuggets of wit and wisdom.

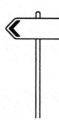

People watching

Ogling people is entirely different from people-watching. The mindful enjoyment of watching others going about their lives can be a great source of pleasure when you're travelling. Just take this advice: don't do it with your mouth open. It's *so* not a good look.

What have you noticed? Who have you noticed? Why did they attract your attention?

Space for more people-watching notes. (If you can, and you're confident you're not risking arrest, draw a picture of the people you're watching here).

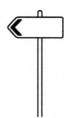

Loves

People commonly fall in love when they're on a trip. It might be with a place, a song, a thing or of course, a person. (It could even be me! No pressure...) What do you love this trip? Why do you love it/them?

More space for more love.

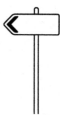

Passions

You may discover a passion for an activity, a sensual pleasure, a place. What arouses strong emotion in you right now? *The stronger the better, baby.*

Why do you feel this way?

Space for raw passion to be expressed in whatever manner you see fit. (You might want to put on some lipstick and kiss the page. Just, you know, suggesting).

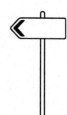

Discoveries

List all the incredible discoveries you're making. It might be how your voice sounds in a cave, how chewing gum tastes when combined with octopus stew, or something about your travel companion you didn't previously know, yet strongly suspected...

Draw a map of all your discoveries. Start with 'Home' and add all the landmarks of your trip to show the path of your journey, your voyage of discovery. Label your discoveries on your map.

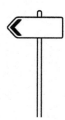

Adrenaline rushes

It could be white-water rafting, hula-hooping, moshing or just feeling suddenly overwhelmingly aware of the miracle of being alive. What's giving you an adrenaline rush on this trip?

More space for more adrenaline rushes.

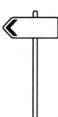

Draw a picture of your face at the height of your biggest adrenaline rush.

Adventures

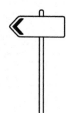

People have different ideas on what constitutes an 'adventure.' An 'adventure' to one person might be an evening filled with knitting and a packet of Snack-a-Jacks. I speak from experience here.

Really though, an adventure is an unusual and possibly dangerous activity that you find exciting. What are your best adventures from this trip? (Note: people can have very different ideas over what 'dangerous' means).

 Further adventures.

Yet more adventures

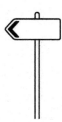

Outstanding beauty

What has really touched your soul this trip? What bowls you over with its majestic, delicate or terrible beauty? (Of course, beauty is always in the eye of the beholder. It isn't always necessarily the guy sitting behind you right now. Although – wow! – just look at him! Ggggrrr).

Why do you find these things so beautiful?

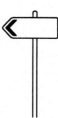

Danger

You may seek danger or you may find yourself suddenly in the midst of it. What are the most dangerous moments of this trip?

Danger! Danger! More space for danger!

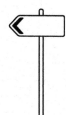

Homesick moments

Sometimes when you're travelling, you might suddenly feel a deep yearning for home. Look at these moments and try to understand what you're actually yearning for. These moments pass although at the time they can be searingly painful. Feel them then let them go. What have you yearned for on this trip?

How have you got through difficult moments?

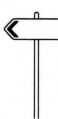

Horrors

Sometimes even the best holidays are marred by horrors. These could be caused by a dodgy burger, a political uprising or plain irresponsible landlords. Write down all your holiday horrors and how you dealt with them here. Honestly, it'll be cathartic.

Proof that things were truly horrible. Stick your proof here.

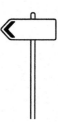

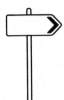

Expectations v Reality

At the start of a holiday expectations are inevitable. What were your expectations at the beginning of this trip?

Have they held up in the face of reality?

How are your expectations changing?

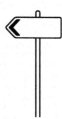

Challenging times

When you're travelling, even the best laid plans can be upset by unexpected events sometimes with tricky logistical consequences. (Think travel delays, missed connecting flights, lost baggage, tears, complaints letters, compensation claims, being featured on a prime time consumer advice programme, getting your own chat show. It happens). What are your challenges? And how are you dealing with them?

More space for notes about challenges. Wipe your tears on this page.

Transport

As you move from one place to the next you'll have to use some kind of transport. What words would you use to describe your experience of transport during this trip?

Wipe this page over the form of transport you've mostly used. Cover it with grime. If the page gets filthy and you've mostly walked, you might consider addressing your personal hygiene.

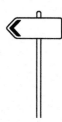

Customs and rituals

These might be the kind of customs the locals perform, it might be your own personal rituals you perform every time you travel... or it might be the kind of customs where you have to declare potentially illegal imports. What are your experiences of customs and rituals on your journey?

How has performing your customs and rituals made you feel?

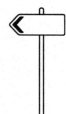

Your companion(s)

Even if you're travelling alone you'll probably have some kind of companion, even if it's only me, your loyal journal. (I promise I won't be offended. I said: **I WON'T BE OFFENDED. NO, REALLY**).

How would you describe your companion(s)? How do you feel about them and their habits?

What are you learning about your companion(s) that you didn't know before the trip?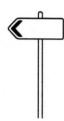

New friends

Even the most casual acquaintance might become a welcome friend when you're on holiday. Who are you meeting who you kinda like?

Why have you connected? What is it about these new friends that you like?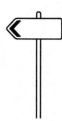

People you contact while you're away

People back home often expect you to contact them while you're travelling; some demand it; some you just want to touch base with; some get **REALLY UPSET** if you don't. Who do you want to contact while you're away? Why? How will you contact them? Phone, email, text, social media?

Space for more thoughts on the folk back home.

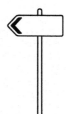

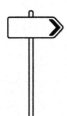

What are you going to tell the people back home about your trip?

Social media updates

Are you tweeting, updating your status or sharing pics while you're away?
With 'beginner's eyes' what can you learn about your social media engagement?

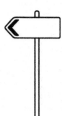

Imagine you're reading your updates as a complete stranger. What perception
would you get of their author?

Write your social media updates here. Stick in pics, if pics are what you've posted.

Wifi codes and techy issues

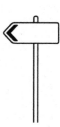

Getting a good signal can make or break a holiday. Oh, the potential heartbreak of not being able to electronically communicate. (This is why an analogue journal is so damn cool!) Write down the wifi codes you need to know here, along with any other techy information that might help.

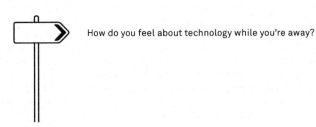

How do you feel about technology while you're away?

Stresses and strains

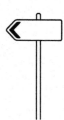

This might mean emotional stress or the physical strain of carrying a backpack (or similar beast) around all the time. How are you coping with stress? Physically? Emotionally? If you're really stressed, try out the mindfulness exercises at the start of this book.

Stuff you packed but don't need

Make a list of everything you really don't need but at the time of packing were convinced you couldn't live without.

What do you notice about your list?

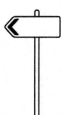

Stuff you wish you'd packed but didn't

And conversely, this is the stuff you really, really miss. Why do you miss it?

What do you notice about this list?

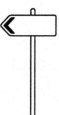

Holiday clothes you haven't worn

Most people (actually, my mother) take loads more clothes away with them than they actually need. Draw them here.

Why aren't you wearing them?

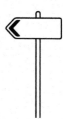

Holiday clothes you wear, like, constantly

Is there a piece of clothing (or several pieces) you find yourself wearing day after day? What do you like about them? How does the fabric, the cut of them feel against your skin?

How do you feel emotionally when you wear these clothes? What are you telling the world about yourself when you wear them?

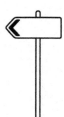

Successful and unsuccessful shoes

Bad shoes can ruin a holiday. Trust me. I know. Write about your shoes and how they helped (or hindered) your mindful walking practice.

Wet the sole of your left foot and stand on this page to make a print of your be-shoed hoof. Or go barefoot if that's your bag.

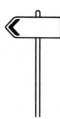

Meditation practice

If you've meditated on this trip, or practiced mindfulness, describe your practice here.

More space for mindful meditation practice notes.

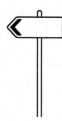

Draw how you feel as a result of your meditation and mindfulness practice.

Leavetaking

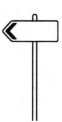

As you leave your temporary holiday home, what are you taking with you... and what are you leaving behind? Literally, metaphorically and spiritually? (Note: this is not in any way a suggestion to steal items from your hotel room. At all).

Stick a brochure, picture or business card here that reminds you of the place you stayed.

Reflecting

Realisations

From time to time we have realisations – the sense of the 'penny dropping' when something that didn't make sense suddenly wonderfully does.
What sudden 'kaboom!' or 'Eureka!' moments are you having as a result of this trip?

Space for more realisations.

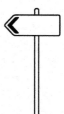

Things you experienced that you wish you hadn't

It might be a very heavy 'morning after the night before,' the clammy kiss of a jellyfish... or the clammy kiss of something altogether more human, but there may be some experiences you may wish you'd not allowed into your life. Purge them here, then let them go. Imagine them sailing off into the sunset, for instance.

Space for notes and drawings about more dodgy experiences. Don't forget to let them go when you're done.

Stuff you now realise you're really grateful for

Going away from home can have the effect of putting things in perspective. Being grateful for things in your life (it could be people, a situation, money, opportunities, food, shelter, water and access to basic medical supplies) can contribute to fostering a positive mindset and a sense of happiness and wellbeing. List the stuff you didn't realise you're thankful for.

More space for your gratitude list.

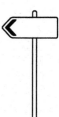

Enduring memories

What are the unforgettable moments of this trip? No matter how much hypnotherapy you have, which memories will you never ever forget?

More unforgettables.

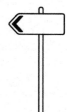

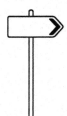

What makes these memories so special to you?

On returning

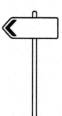

When you return, what's the first thing you notice about your home? Why is that the first thing you notice?

What's changed about your home, both inside and outside?

Stuff you learned

Popular wisdom says that travel broadens the mind, so how has your mind
been expanded? It might be factual things, profound things, stuff about people
or stuff about you.

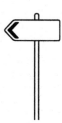

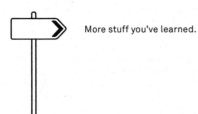 More stuff you've learned.

People you wish you'd brought with you

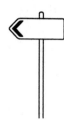

If you'd had the opportunity, who would you have asked to join you on your trip? Why them? Why now?

What stopped you from asking them to go with you?

People you wish you'd left at home

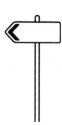

Sometimes our relationships with our travel companions can be sorely challenged during a trip. If your relationships have changed as a result of your holiday, what's caused that? How do you feel about it?

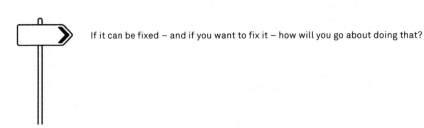

If it can be fixed – and if you want to fix it – how will you go about doing that?

Things, places, people, food etc that you want to experience again

Here's an opportunity to relive parts of your trip again, albeit in a different setting, time and place. Make a list of everything you want to do again. And again. And again. Think about why you enjoy them so much.

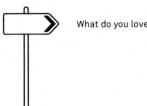

What do you love about these experiences?

Things you enjoy more in retrospect

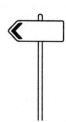

It might be trekking through a swamp, going on a roller coaster, eating squid – sometimes there are things we do on holiday that at the time seem truly awful but we enjoy later, through our memories. Which bits of your trip will you enjoy more through the lens of nostalgia?

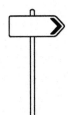 More space for retrospective enjoyment

Peace

Sometimes on our travels away from the hustle and bustle we have special moments of peace and serenity. Remember the moment you felt most at peace and write three or four words to describe this moment. Now draw a simple symbol, a doodle, or whatever you like to depict that moment, that peaceful feeling. Writing and drawing this will help bring back those feelings when you need them.

Wish-list for your next trip

This holiday might be over, but that's no reason to get out of holiday-mode completely. Plan your next trip here. Where to go, what to do...what not to do. All that your holiday heart desires. You get the gist.

Random thoughts

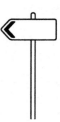

 More random thoughts

The more random the better

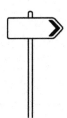 That's it! Now for the **really** random stuff...

It's time to stop. Or is it??

I am complete, finished and utterly done. My pages are stuffed with smells, objects, memories, hopes, dreams and many, many stains. Just flick through the pages now. Go on.

Wow.

That felt good, didn't it??

Your moments are splurged, etched, and stuck to my pages. I contain the life you've lived during your holiday.

Imagine: in many years from now, someone may find me sitting on a shelf - a future film director, a novelist, a poet, a grand child. Blowing away the dust, they see the journey we've taken together, our unique moments that belong to another time. And they're enchanted not because you wrestled crocodiles in the Amazon (unless you actually did - in which case: WOW!) but because this story has been told through your unique eyes.

It's been a privilege. Really. Thank you for trusting me to be the custodian of your precious memories.

Now, let's stop this. I'm hopeless at goodbyes.

Just don't be a stranger, OK?

By the way, there are other Sit.Breathe.Love. journals available on our website.

It really doesn't have to stop here, you know...

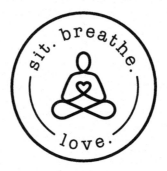

Ready to order your next Journal?

Just go to SitBreatheLove.com and order your copy.

We sincerely hope you've enjoyed your journal. Let us know how you used it – we love getting feedback.

Check out our website too. We have a bunch of free stuff, including some meditations.

Email: hello@sitbreathelove.com

Follow: @SitBreatheLove

Acknowledgments

Big thanks to David Birtles, Simon Galloway, Alison Metcalfe, Shelly Smith, Rich Sweetman (whose Asian odyssey led me to think about writing a mindful travel journal), Kirsty Galloway, Neil Kerfoot, Matt Haworth, James Hanson, Julia Brosnan, Grant Appleton and a special thanks to Becky Perry.

About the author

Emma Clarke is a writer and broadcaster. She's been practicing mindfulness since 1999. She lives in Manchester with her husband and two children.

EmmaClarke.com   @emmabclarke

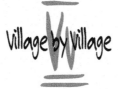

Village by Village – Who We Are

Village by Village was established in 2006 after the founder witnessed the implication of a lack of clean water, sanitation and education in remote disadvantaged rural communities in Ghana. The charity was established to respond to the needs of these communities by supporting the reduction of poverty and needless hygiene-related deaths through the provision of simple but powerful resources and opportunities.

Since 2006 projects established have provided toilets, clean drinking water, scholarship programmes to enable children to attend school and support for individuals to start up their own businesses. The charity has grown to a team of 10 dedicated staff, nine of whom are based in country. We work in partnership with those people living in poverty in the rural villages as we have found this provides the greatest impact. Through this way of working, Ghanaian based project contractors and volunteers have established solid partnerships and so work in collaboration to best deliver the projects, adding value to the work of others operating in Ghana.

Impact to Date

Our original aim was to reach 100 villages by 2016 with sanitation, clean drinking water education for children and business skills. We were able to reach this aim by February 2012 four years ahead of schedule due to the effectiveness of the partnership working with community members in the villages in Ghana which included the incorporation of community ideas and knowledge and the employment and engagement of those within the communities.

Through our work we have supported approximately 35,000 people in 100 villages to reduce poverty and to improve their self-sustainability, health and life chances. Since 2006 we have delivered:

- Completed 36 toilet projects in communities and schools to help reduce deaths due to poor sanitation
- 4 wells built to provide clean drinking water in villages
- 2 rain water harvesting projects for hand washing projects in schools in communities in poverty
- 711 children provided with the opportunity to educate their way out of poverty through the provision of scholarships
- 6 businesses developed to support sustainable incomes
- A health clinic was built in Gboloo, Kofi which has been staffed by the local health service
- A school library and information centre was established to provide information on health, hygiene, sanitation and family planning to the remote villages surrounding Gboloo, Kofi
- Built a crèche and kindergarten allowing very young children to access a village school
- Built a Junior High School in the remote rural village of Gboloo Kofi
- Built a Primary School block and computer lab in the remote rural village of Abenta

The Need — Preventable Death

Having spent six years working alongside communities in poverty working together to provide sanitation projects Village by Village have found the biggest impact in saving the lives of children and reducing pain and suffering amongst families does not simply come from providing toilets and wells, but must be combined with teaching the importance of washing hands with soap.

Diarrhoeal disease remains one of the world's biggest killers, with UNICEF estimating it kills a child every 30 seconds. In Ghana, diarrhoea accounts for 25 percent of all deaths in children under five and is among the top three reported causes of deaths.

While hand-washing in the UK may help prevent a stomach bug, in poorer countries it is the most effective and in-expensive way to save lives. Without ready access to hand washing facilities including running water and soap, coupled with an understanding of its importance, entire communities will remain at risk. Turning hand washing with soap before and after eating and using the toilet into an ingrained habit could save more lives than any single vaccine or medical intervention, cutting deaths from diarrhoea by almost half and deaths from acute respiratory infections by one-quarter.

Village by Village have witnessed the impact of poor sanitation first hand though our 100 Village's project. This project offered toilets and hand washing facilities to households and communities as a whole.

It is now our priority to establish the importance of sanitation throughout those communities we have worked in, to ensure further lives are not unnecessarily lost.

The Solution – Clean Hands Saves Lives, an integrated approach

To improve the life chances of some of the most vulnerable individuals and communities within Ghana our 'Clean Hands Saves Lives' project will provide sanitation facilities whilst also addressing behavioural change to support a life-time impact.

During 2012-16 we will target 5,600 children aged 6-16 with the facilities, resources and education to ingrain the washing of hands following toilet use. Children are strategically being targeted to provide the greatest impact as not only do they suffer disproportionally from diarrhoeal diseases, it has been proven that once children change their behaviour, 80 percent are then likely to pass their learning to their own families.

To ensure the necessary change takes place to improve health and life chances, the project will be implemented within two separate phases:

1. **Providing the tools**

   Each project will begin with the help of our local & international volunteers who work alongside our team of Ghanaian builders to build a three toilet, block within a schools. These toilet blocks support sanitation as their self composting design ensures flies entering the toilet are trapped inside the pit latrine. Their larvae developed into maggots which eat away the faeces.

   Polytanks (plastic water tanks) and guttering is used to collect rainwater that will support hand washing. With the use of a veronica bucket (a plastic container designed with a tap at the bottom, see the photo to the right) water is released into a bowl acting as a sink. All equipment can be locally replaced and repaired increase the longevity of the project. Soap will be provided by the school as a sign of their commitment before a school is selected.

2. Behaviour Change

Once the necessary tools have been provided, an intensive supporting phase will commence over a 18 month period. This will establish new patterns of behaviour to embed hand-washing to improve sanitation. The Ghana Health Service and the Education Service will join the project at this stage, providing teachers and nurses to talk to the local scholl children alongside headteachers who will engage village Chiefs and Elders who will support the community wide message and enhance commitment to the project. We provide the teachers and children with promotional materials to incentive. reward and encourage behaviour change, including t-shirts, stickers, posters and baseball caps.

Once the community is engaged, the children will be targeted through a 'Bog Watch' initiative. This will act as an engagement tool with volunteers recruited as behavioural change agents. As recommended by the local headteachers consulted, a rota system will be put into place to encourage hand-washing with classmates acting as hand-washing monitors. Teams of school children will be tasked with designing and brightly painting the toilet blocks and water tanks with promotional hand-washing messages aimed at their classmates.

To further enhance commitment to the project, children and members of the local community will be chosen as 'star' actors to appear in a hand washing flash-mob film. This is screened as a whole community movie-night using a projector and a white sheet.

This creates an exciting and memorable experience for the community as a whole as such events are very rarely held. An example of a film made can be found at: **www.youtube.com/watchv=YGhqok0wBGE**

Monitoring and Evaluation

We will put in place a comprehensive monitoring and evaluation system to measure the impact of the project. This will include the following:

- A baseline survey with regular surveys thereafter recording the outputs and the impact of the project.

The following will also be implemented as an engagement opportunity, however the data collected will also be used within the monitoring process over the 18 month period:

- Playground surveys conducted by the children
- Child centric and adult centric 'bog watch' carried out by school children / members of the community assessing the number of people washing their hands following visits to the toilet.

How to donate

With your support we hope to continue to make a difference to some of the poorest communities in Ghana, improving health and saving lives.

To donate to Village by Village, just click: **www.sitbreathelove.com/donate**